Health Financing Strategy for the Asia Pacific Region (2010-2015)

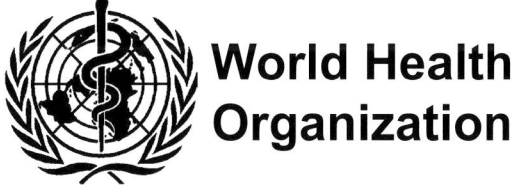

World Health Organization

South-East Asia Region   Western Pacific Region

WHO Library Cataloguing in Publication Data

Health financing strategy for the Asia Pacific region (2010-2015).

1. Delivery of health care – economics. 2. Health services – economics. 3. Health care economics and organizations. 4. Financing, Government. 5. Asia and the Pacific.

ISBN 978-92-9061-458-6   (NLM Classification: WA 525)

© World Health Organization 2009

All rights reserved. Publications of the World Health Organization can be obtained from WHO Press, World Health Organization, 20 Avenue Appia, 1211 Geneva 27, Switzerland (tel.: +41 22 791 3264; fax: +41 22 791 4857; e-mail: bookorders@who.int). Requests for permission to reproduce or translate WHO publications – whether for sale or for noncommercial distribution – should be addressed to WHO Press, at the above address (fax: +41 22 791 4806; e-mail: permissions@who.int).   For WHO Western Pacific Regional Publications, request for permission to reproduce should be addressed to the Publications Office, World Health Organization, Regional Office for the Western Pacific, P.O. Box 2932, 1000, Manila, Philippines, Fax. No. (632) 521-1036, email: publications@wpro.who.int

The designations employed and the presentation of the material in this publication do not imply the expression of any opinion whatsoever on the part of the World Health Organization concerning the legal status of any country, territory, city or area or of its authorities, or concerning the delimitation of its frontiers or boundaries. Dotted lines on maps represent approximate border lines for which there may not yet be full agreement.

The mention of specific companies or of certain manufacturers' products does not imply that they are endorsed or recommended by the World Health Organization in preference to others of a similar nature that are not mentioned. Errors and omissions excepted, the names of proprietary products are distinguished by initial capital letters.

All reasonable precautions have been taken by the World Health Organization to verify the information contained in this publication. However, the published material is being distributed without warranty of any kind, either expressed or implied. The responsibility for the interpretation and use of the material lies with the reader. In no event shall the World Health Organization be liable for damages arising from its use.

Table of contents

	page
Executive Summary	v

1. Introduction 1
   1.1 900 million vulnerable to impoverishment from health care costs 1
   1.2 The global recession and health 2
   1.3 Rationale for updating the health financing strategy 2

2. Health financing issues in the Asia Pacific region 5
   2.1 Sources of financing and out-of-pocket expenditures 5
   2.2 Efficiency issues in the Region 11

3. Health financing for universal coverage 17
   3.1 Universal coverage is difficult to achieve if out-of-pocket payments >30% of THE 17
   3.2 Universal coverage is difficult to achieve if public financing is less than 5% of GDP 18
   3.3 Fiscal space, aid effectiveness, and efficiency gains 19
   3.4 Health systems strengthening and health financing 22

4. Health Financing Strategy for the Asia Pacific Region (2010–2015) 25
   4.1 Advancing towards universal coverage 25
   4.2 Goals and targets 26
   4.3 Supportive environment for health financing reforms ..28
   4.4 Strategic areas for action in health financing for universal coverage 29

5. Conclusions 37
   Health Financing Strategy Glossary 39

List of figures

Figure 1   Sources of health expenditure by region 6

Figure 2   Improverishment and catastrophic expenses due to health care costs by WHO region 7

Figure 3   Percentage of GDP of government and private health spending and total expenditure in the Asia Pacific region 8

Figure 4   Private health expenditures vs. government health spending in South-East Asia and Western Pacific countries (2007) 8

Figure 5   Social health insurance coverage vs. social health insurance expenditures (2006) 11

Figure 6   Allocation of financial resources to primary health care (2005 estimates) 12

Figure 7   Components of health expenditure (2005) 15

Figure 8   Components of health expenditure (2005) 16

Figure 9   Percentage of households with catastrophic expenditures vs. share of out-of-pocket payment in total health expenditure 20

Figure 10   Percentage of households with catastrophic expenditures vs. government health expenditures as a share of GDP 20

Figure 11   Health systems framework with six building blocks 22

Figure 12   Attainment of universal coverage 25

Figure 13   Steps towards universal coverage 26

Figure 14   Links between health financing strategy and health outcomes 27

List of tables

Table 1   Asia Pacific countries grouped by level of total health expenditure (2007) 9

Table 2   Main provider payment methods in the Western Pacific Region 14

Executive summary

Universal coverage and access to quality health services to achieve better health outcomes are widely recognized goals in the Asia Pacific region, which includes the 37 countries and areas of the WHO Western Pacific Region and the 11 countries of the WHO South-East Asia Region. Member States in the region are at various stages of progress towards these goals. In response to changes in socioeconomic conditions and the global health environment, WHO is updating its regional health financing strategy to better support universal coverage.

The global economic downturn poses challenges as well as opportunities to improve health systems financing in the region. The current economic difficulties are further burdening stressed health care budgets and are placing millions of people at risk of greater impoverishment due to health care expenses or ill-health due to inadequate health care. Current levels of out-of-pocket health spending in the Asia Pacific region are much higher than in other parts of the world. A strong and informed government role is needed in the provision, regulation and financing of health systems. A reduction in out-of-pocket payments is a necessary condition to move towards universal coverage. Global evidence indicates that it is difficult to achieve universal coverage and high financial protection if out-of-pocket payments are higher than 30% of total health expenditures.

The level of government spending on health is too low in many countries in the region to support universal coverage. Governments are encouraged to develop strategies to increase investments and public spending on health. At the same time, actions to improve efficiency in the use of available public financial resources for health are needed.

There is a renewed global and regional focus on health systems based on the principles and values of primary health care, particularly the value of equity. Many health systems have invested heavily in curative services and have spent relatively less on preventive, promotive and primary health care services. The call for universal coverage based on the principles of primary health care has encouraged a policy dialogue on national health financing policies and plans to build more equitable, efficient and effective health systems.

The Health Financing Strategy for the Asia Pacific Region (2010–2015) will help governments analyse their health financing situations and identify specific actions to achieve universal coverage. It was developed as a result of regional health financing reviews and consultations and is based on a growing body of global research and evidence.

Universal coverage usually is attained in countries in which public financing of health is around 5% of gross domestic product (GDP). This is an important goal for all countries in the Asia Pacific region to consider as they move towards universal coverage. However, there is considerable variation among countries. The updated Strategy encourages countries to set their own realistic targets, with a clear strategic course of action to increase public spending and the government share of total health expenditures. This will enable the expansion of financing from prepaid and risk-pooled sources, thus reducing out-of-pocket expenditures. It will also have impacts on population coverage and social health protection, which will benefit the poor and vulnerable.

The following target indicators are proposed to monitor and evaluate overall progress in attaining universal coverage in countries and in the Asia Pacific region:

(1) out-of-pocket spending should not exceed 30%–40% of total health expenditure;
(2) total health expenditure should be at least 4%–5% of the gross domestic product;
(3) over 90% of the population is covered by prepayment and risk-pooling schemes; and
(4) close to 100% coverage of vulnerable populations with social assistance and safety-net programmes.

The updated Strategy maintains five of the strategic areas from the current Strategy on Health Care Financing for Countries of the Western Pacific and South-East Asia Regions (2006-2010). In addition, it adds three new areas intended to improve aid effectiveness, more efficiently use resources and improve provider payment methods. The eight strategic areas are:

(1) increasing investment and public spending on health
(2) improving aid effectiveness for health
(3) improving efficiency by rationalizing health expenditures
(4) increasing the use of prepayment and pooling
(5) improving provider payment methods
(6) strengthening safety-net mechanisms for the poor and vulnerable
(7) improving evidence and information for policymaking, and
(8) improving monitoring and evaluation of policy changes.

Each of the eight areas contains core strategic actions that can be modified according to country conditions and needs. All contribute to attaining universal coverage of quality health services. The implementation of the Strategy may require health financing reform. Such reforms require consensus- based commitment, improved national capacities, transparent and accountable decision-making, and monitoring and evaluation of universal coverage policy and regulations. WHO is committed to supporting universal coverage in all Member States and helping build more equitable, efficient and effective health systems to achieve the highest attainable levels of health for the people of the Asia Pacific region.

1. Introduction

Improved health is the overarching public health policy objective across the Asia Pacific region. Health status has improved greatly in many countries, particularly those where governments are committed to universal coverage of health services based on the values and principles of primary health care, but much remains to be done. The promotion of health equity through universal coverage is one of four areas of health systems reform that supports people-centered health services and the renewal of primary health care.[1] Reforms in service delivery, public policy and leadership are also essential to promote and protect the health of communities and part of the renewed focus on primary health care.

The WHO framework for health systems strengthening Everybody's business: Strengthening health systems to improve health outcomes. provides a platform for analysis using six health systems building blocks to design integrated action to achieve improved health outcomes.[2] The sixty-first session of the WHO Regional Committee for South-East Asia and the fifty-ninth session of the WHO Regional Committee for the Western Pacific endorsed independent resolutions to strengthen health systems based on the values and principles of primary health care.[3,4] Universal access to or coverage by quality health services without excessive household financial burden is the overarching goal.

1.1 900 million vulnerable to impoverishment from health care costs

Economic development in the Asia Pacific region has lifted millions out of poverty. However, 900 million people still subsist on less than US$ 2 a day. The relationship between good health and economic development is well accepted. The United Nations Millennium Development Goals focus much attention on

---

[1] *The World Health Report 2008. Primary Health Care, Now More Than Ever.*
[2] *Everybody's business. Strengthening health systems to improve health outcomes. WHO's framework for action. WHO 2007.*
[3] *Regional Committee resolution SEAR/RC61/R3.*
[4] *Regional Committee resolution WPR/RC59.R4.*

improving health status and reducing poverty. Health systems that provide universal coverage and affordable access to the poor and disadvantaged both improve health and fight poverty. The lack of financial risk protection from health care costs drives millions into poverty as they struggle to pay for health care. It also drives millions away from needed health care due to inability to pay and fear of catastrophic expenditure.

1.2 The global recession and health

The current global economic downturn is creating new challenges, and results will vary. Countries that rely heavily on exports of raw or manufactured products will experience job losses and internal migration. In other countries, remittances from overseas workers may be reduced. Social needs are likely to grow, while government commitments to health may be reduced because of decreasing revenues. Unemployment will also reduce funds for all types of social insurance. Countries may be tempted to reduce their social safety nets and preventive health programmes. As financial protection for health is reduced and people begin to save more money due to the uncertain economic times, domestic consumption could decrease and impede economic recovery. Donor countries may also reduce overseas development assistance.

1.3 Rationale for updating the health financing strategy

The current Strategy on Health Care Financing for Countries of the Western Pacific and South-East Asia Regions (2006–2010) was endorsed by the Regional Committee at its fifty-sixth session in September 2005. A midterm review of the Strategy indicated that progress towards achieving universal coverage and access to quality health services need further support and advocacy in the region. The recent focus on health systems strengthening and primary health care renewal highlighted the crucial role of health care financing in building equitable and efficient health systems. The international community has increased donor assistance in health. Donor assistance is most effectively used if it is part of a comprehensive health financing framework. In addition, the current economic crisis increases the need for public intervention and financing of essential health services and social safety nets, especially for the poor and vulnerable. These changes indicate a need to update the health financing strategy. The draft Health Financing Strategy for the Asia Pacific Region (2010–2015) is based on findings obtained in the midterm review of countries and areas in the Western Pacific Region,[5] the experience and perspectives of countries in the South-East Asia Region, and the ever increasing body of global evidence. The updated Strategy maintains five of the seven strategic areas from the 2006–2010 document, while adding three new strategic areas to align with evolving regional priorities and changing economic conditions.

The main objective is universal coverage. Substantial evidence exists that universal coverage can be achieved when governments take strong and informed roles in the provision, regulation and financing of health systems, and maintain a clear focus on primary health care. WHO is committed to supporting its Member States in moving towards these objectives.

---

[5]Mid-term review of implementation: Regional Strategy on Health Care Financing in the WHO Western Pacific Region 2006-2010. 31 August 2008.

2. Health financing issues in Asia and the Pacific

In 2008, the WHO Regional Office for the Western Pacific commissioned a 14-country midterm review of the implementation of the Strategy on Health Care Financing for Countries of the Western Pacific and South-East Asia Regions (2006–2010). In early 2009, the WHO Regional Office for South-East Asia reviewed country experiences in its Region at a seminar on health financing. A draft updated health financing strategy was prepared, and in March 2009 a panel of experts from all WHO regions and most major donor organizations reviewed the draft strategy and proposed revisions. The revised draft was further reviewed at a second meeting in Manila in April 2009, with participants from 13 Member States in the South-East Asia and Western Pacific Regions. Their input is reflected in the current WHO framework for action for strengthening health systems. Major health care financing issues are discussed below.

2.1 Sources of financing and out-of-pocket expenditures

Levels of private out-of-pocket (OOP) health spending in the Asia Pacific region are much higher than other regions, making up over 40% of total health expenditures (THE) in the Western Pacific Region and over 60% in the South-East Asia Region (Figure 1).

Absolute levels of catastrophic payments and impoverishment due to health care costs in the region are among the highest in the world (Figure 2). In 2005, an estimated 80 million people faced catastrophic health expenses, and 50 million people were impoverished because of out-of-pocket payments associated with poor health status and use of health services. Rates of impoverishment due to health care costs in China and Viet Nam are among the highest in the world. Catastrophic health care costs pushed an estimated 39.5 million people in India below the poverty line in one year.[6] The current

---

[6]Bonu, S. I. Bhushan, and D. Peters. 2007. Incidence, Intensity, and Correlates of Catastrophic Out-of-Pocket Health Payments in India. Economics and Research Department Working Papers Series 102. ADB Manila.

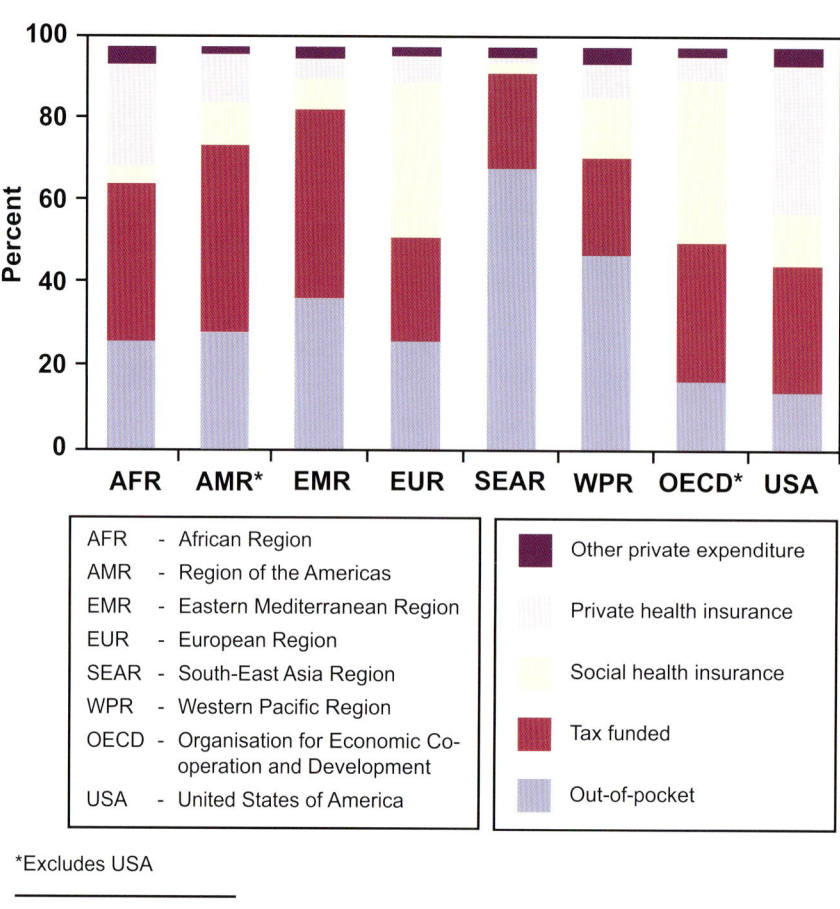

Figure 1. Sources of health expenditure by region (2005)

*Excludes USA

Source: WHO/EIP/HSF/CEP

economic crisis may increase vulnerability substantially unless governments protect social spending and improve social health protection measures.

National health accounts data for 2007 shows that government spending on health in most developing countries in the Asia Pacific region is below 5% of GDP and less than 2% in nearly half of them (Figure 3).

Out-of-pocket payments are the largest source of health care financing in most countries, especially those with low levels of government expenditure on health. Countries with less than 2% government spending have exceptionally high private health expenditures (Figure 4). Most countries in the region with government spending on health of greater than 5% of GDP have less

Figure 2. Improverishment and catastrophic expenses due to health care costs by WHO region

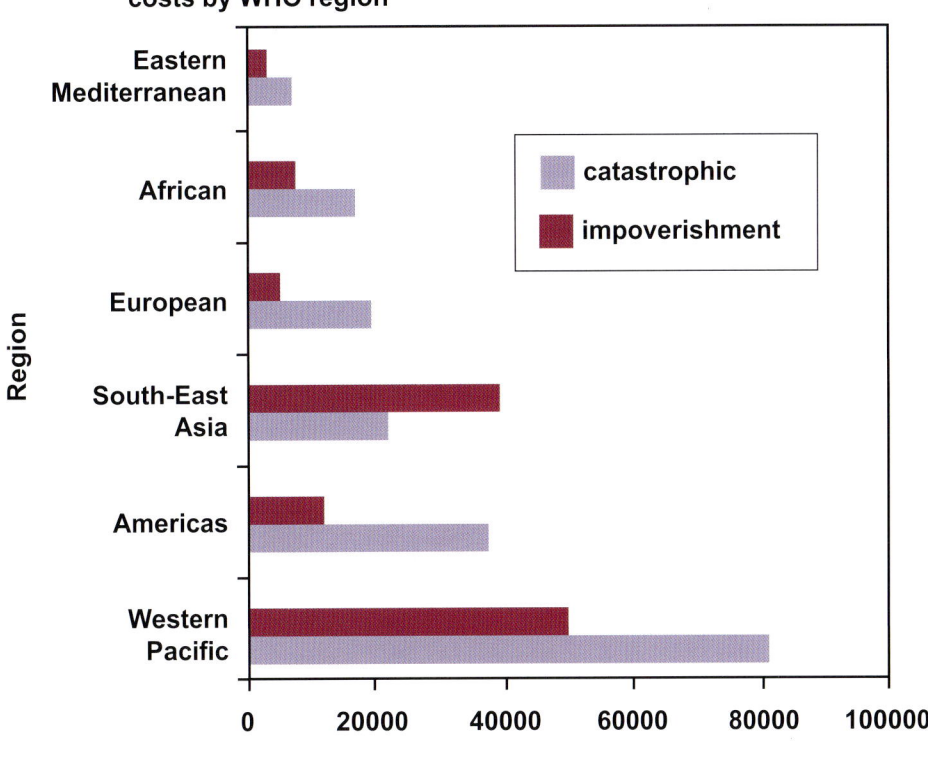

Source: K Xu, D Evans, G Carrin, A Aguilar, P Musgrove, T Evans. (2007). Protecting Households from Catastrophic Health Spending. Health Affairs, 26, no.4 (2007): 972-983

than 30% out-of-pocket health expenditures. This relationship is also seen globally.

The share of government health expenditure in total health spending is an important indicator of government commitment to health. Despite increases in several countries over the 2005–2007 period, government spending was less than half of total health expenditures in 16 out of 48 countries and areas of the Asia Pacific region, including nearly all the most populous countries, and below 40% in Bangladesh, Cambodia, India, the Lao People's Democratic Republic, Myanmar and the Philippines.

While government health spending in the region is low, even the addition of private spending brings the total health expenditure to less than 5% of GDP in 19 out of the 48 countries and areas in the two WHO regions that make

Figure 3. Percentage of GDP of government and private health spending and total expenditure in the Asia Pacific region

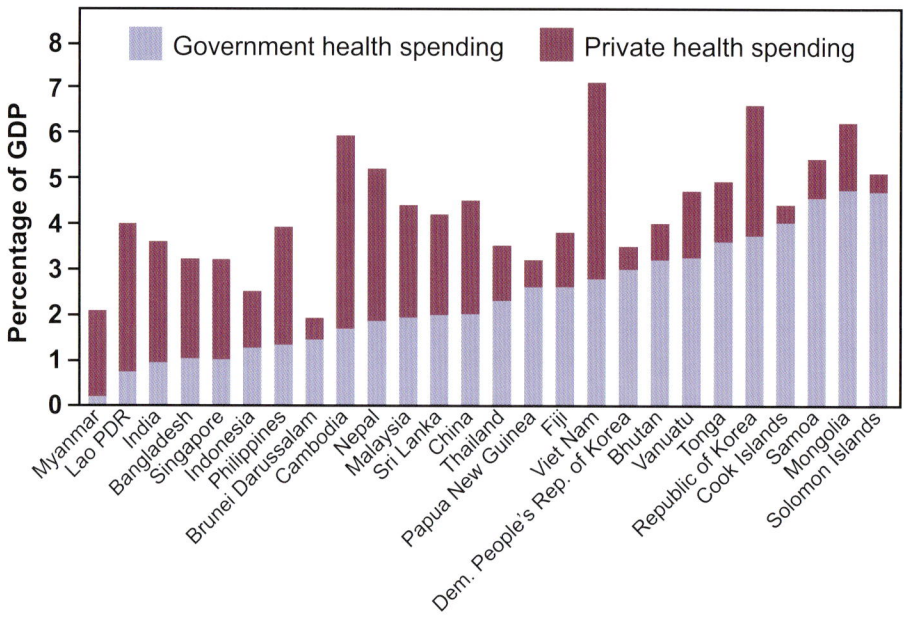

Source: WHO Provisional 2007 NHA data

Figure 4. Private health expenditures vs. government health spending in South-East Asia and Western Pacific countries (2007)

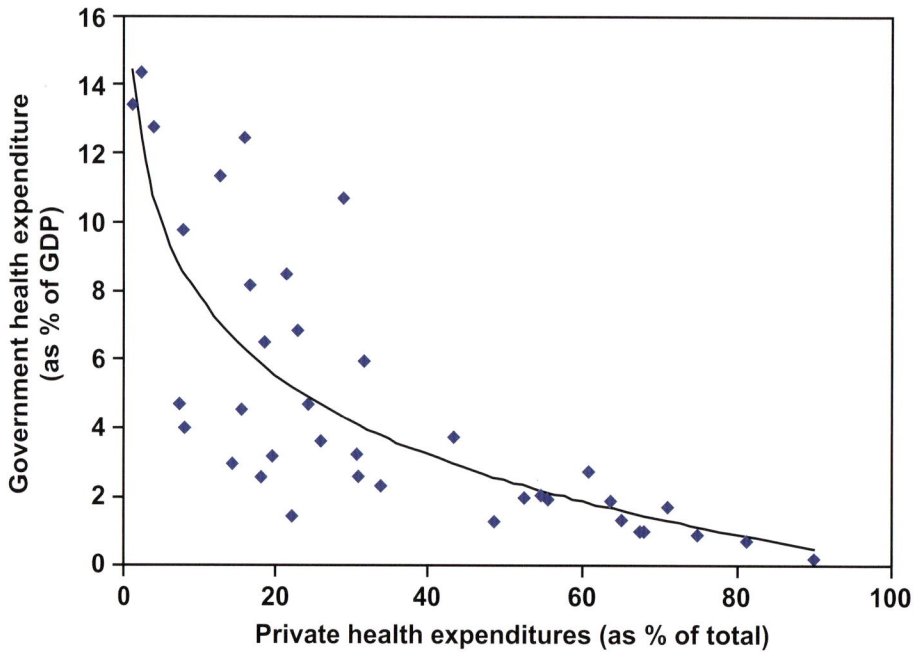

Source: Provisional NHA data 2007

up the larger Asia Pacific region (Table 1). Wealthier countries, such as Brunei Darussalam, Malaysia and Singapore, nevertheless provide comprehensive quality care with universal access because of their higher per capita GDP, with total per capita health expenditures near or above US$ 500. Malaysia also provides effective social safety nets.

Per capita health spending (at average exchange rates) is still less than the WHO Commission on Macroeconomics and Health benchmark of US$ 35 in five countries, and below $100 in 15 out of the 48 countries and areas in the Asia Pacific region.

Table 1   Asia Pacific countries grouped by level of total health expenditure (2007)

Total health expenditure of Asia-Pacific countries as % of GDP		
Below 5%	Between 5%–7%	Above 7%
Bangladesh Bhutan Brunei Darussalam China Cook Islands Democratic People's Republic of Korea Fiji India Indonesia Lao People's Democratic Republic Malaysia Myanmar Papua New Guinea Philippines Sri Lanka Thailand Singapore Tonga Vanuatu	Cambodia Mongolia Nepal Republic of Korea Samoa Solomon Islands	Australia Japan Kiribati Marshall Islands Micronesia, Federated States of Maldives Nauru New Zealand Niue Palau Timor-Leste Tuvalu Viet Nam

Source: NHA data estimates, WHO 2007.

Some governments reduced out-of-pocket payments between 2005 and 2007. For example, out-of-pocket payments as a percentage of total health expenditures fell from 54% to 49% in China, from 37% to 28% in Mongolia, and from 67% to 62% in Viet Nam. The main reasons were the expansion of coverage by rural and urban insurance schemes in China, increased allocation of the government budget to health in Mongolia, and public subsidy for social health insurance premiums for the poor in Viet Nam.

In China, health insurance coverage increased from 23% of the population in 2005 to 80% in 2007, with the government-sponsored Rural Cooperative Medical System alone covering 842 million people.[7] Population insurance coverage also increased in the same period from 55% to 77% in the Philippines and from 34% to 42% in Viet Nam. Population coverage increased in the Lao People's Democratic Republic, largely from government-sponsored, community-based health insurance schemes. While some countries with high informal and subsistence farming employment are just beginning to cover their populations by social health insurance (SHI), Mongolia is now trying to reach the remaining 20% of the population who are not registered for the premium subsidy.

In China, the Philippines and Viet Nam, financial protection has a fairly wide breadth of coverage, but the depth of coverage is low (Figure 5). The limited financial protection granted by some SHI schemes is due to requirements for payment of an "excess" or "deductible" payment and caps on total reimbursements. It was estimated that SHI in China reimburses on average only 30%–40% of patient hospital costs. Only the wealthier insured who can afford these high co-payments have access.

In addition to low effective access, retrospective reimbursement payments used by some SHI schemes are inefficient and costly, thereby inhibiting uptake of insurance benefits and interfering with effective purchasing of services. Multiple insurance schemes with different co-payments and benefit packages can also deter utilization.

---

[7]Shanlian Hu, Universal coverage and health financing from China's perspective. Bull. of the WHO, November 2008, 86 (11)

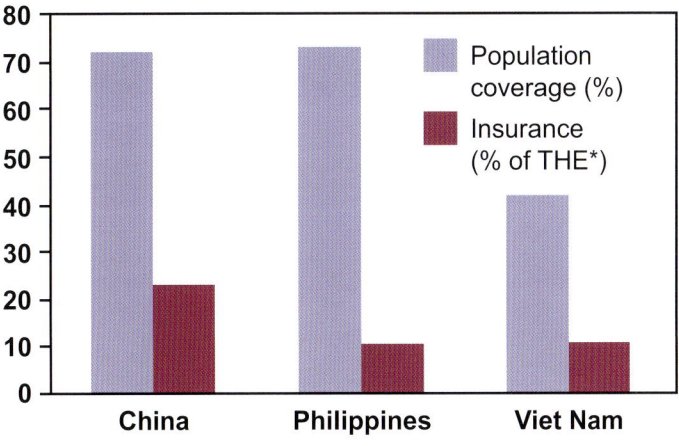

Figure 5. Social health insurance coverage vs. social health insurance expenditures (2006)

Source: 2006 NHA data
*THE = Total health expenditure

Some countries have focused on improving the effectiveness of safety net mechanisms. In China, the New Cooperative Medical Services now has the ability to use a fund from the Ministry of Welfare to pay premiums of people who cannot afford them. In Cambodia, Health Equity Funds target external resources to subsidize hospital expenses of the poor. Viet Nam has a subsidy scheme that covers most of the poor with social health insurance.

2.2 Efficiency issues in the Asia Pacific region

The midterm review found that local improvements in technical and allocative efficiency are needed and feasible. Perhaps 80% of essential care and 70% of desirable health interventions can be delivered at the primary level, but an average of only 10% of health resources are used for primary level care in Asia.[8] The midterm review found that six countries in the Asia Pacific region spent less than 20% on primary health care (Figure 6). By comparison, in 11 OECD countries, outpatient care costs averaged 28% of total health expenditure.

---

[8] *Health Sector reform in Asia and the Pacific: Options for Developing Countries.* ADB, 1999

Figure 6. Allocation of financial resources to primary health care. (2005 estimates)

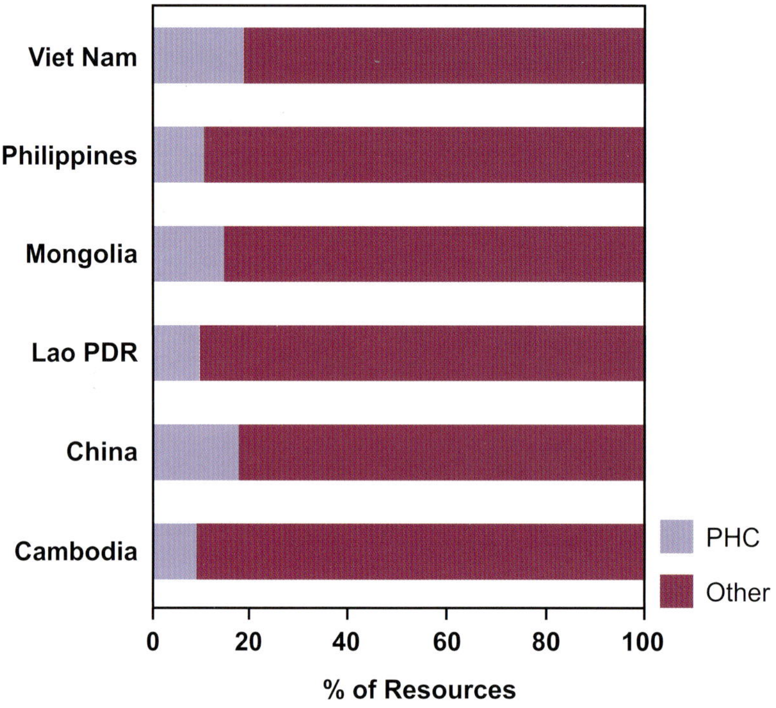

Source: Midterm review of implementation: Regional Strategy on Health Care Financing in the WHO Western Pacific Region 2006-2010, P. Annear, 31 August 2008

Cambodia plans to increase its government budget spending and align it with donor funding to improve efficiency and effectiveness of service delivery. Analytical tools have been used in Cambodia and China to prioritize maternal and child health interventions. The Philippines' health sector reform agenda sets targets that increase the allocation of resources to public health from 11% to 20% and reduce hospital-based personal health care costs from 79% to 62% by 2010.[9] The health sector strategic master plan of Mongolia prioritizes increasing government participation and financial support of preventive and promotive activities.[10]

---

[9] Health Sector Reform Agenda, Philippines, 2006.
[10] Health Sector Strategic Master Plan, 2006-2015. Government of Mongolia, 2005

Reprioritizing preventive care for chronic diseases has the potential for large savings, but governments must take the initiative. More than 90% of diabetes-related expenses in several Pacific island countries were for management and treatment of complications, rather than the more cost-effective early detection and secondary prevention.[11]

The main provider payment methods in the Asia Pacific region are budget allocations, staff salaries and fees for services (Table 2). All countries studied in the midterm review use various fees for services, and in general are inadequately regulated and monitored. Fee-for-service provider payments create perverse incentives for providers to generate income by increasing the volume of profitable services and products, such as advanced diagnostics and pharmaceuticals.[12] More efficient modes of provider payment, such as capitation, are used in Thailand and many OECD countries.[13]

Public spending on the health workforce is relatively low in the continental Asian countries studied. The share of salaries in total health expenditures was only 15% in Cambodia, 17% in Viet Nam and 18% in the Lao People's Democratic Republic (Figure 7), although health worker remuneration paid through fees for service is not captured. The review found that the problem of out-of-pocket payments was most serious when salary levels failed to meet basic needs of health workers. Low budgetary spending on compensation of health professionals encouraged government staff to have private practices and led to poorly regulated user fees in public health facilities.

It was reported that some public hospitals in China received only about 30% of their revenues from the Government, requiring them to generate the rest from other sources including user fees, drugs and diagnostic procedures.[14] While there is willingness among some individuals to pay for these products,

---

[11] Diabetes and the Care Continuum in the Pacific Island Countries. Health Care Decision-making in the Western Pacific Region, WHO/WPRO 2003.

[12] *The work of WHO in the Western Pacific. Report of the Regional Director (1 July 2001–30 June 2002).* WHO, Manila, 2002.

[13] Provider Payments and cost-containment – Lessons from OECD countries. Technical Briefs for Policy-Makers Number 2 2007. WHO/HSF/HFP

[14] Qingyue Meng et al. The impact of China's retail drug price control policy on hospital expenditure. Health Policy and Planning 20(3):185-196 2005; Oxford University Press.

Table 2. Main provider payment methods in the Asia Pacific Region

Budgets/salary	Fee for service	Capitation/ case payment/ diagnostic-related groups	Mixed
Bhutan Brunei Darussalam Cook Islands Democratic People's Republic of Korea Fiji Kiribati Maldives Marshall Islands Micronesia, Federated States of Nauru Niue Palau Papua New Guinea Samoa Solomon Islands Timor-Leste Tuvalu Tonga Vanuatu	Bangladesh Cambodia China India Lao People's Democratic Republic Myanmar Nepal Viet Nam	Australia New Zealand	Indonesia Japan Malaysia, Mongolia Philippines Republic of Korea Singapore Sri Lanka Thailand

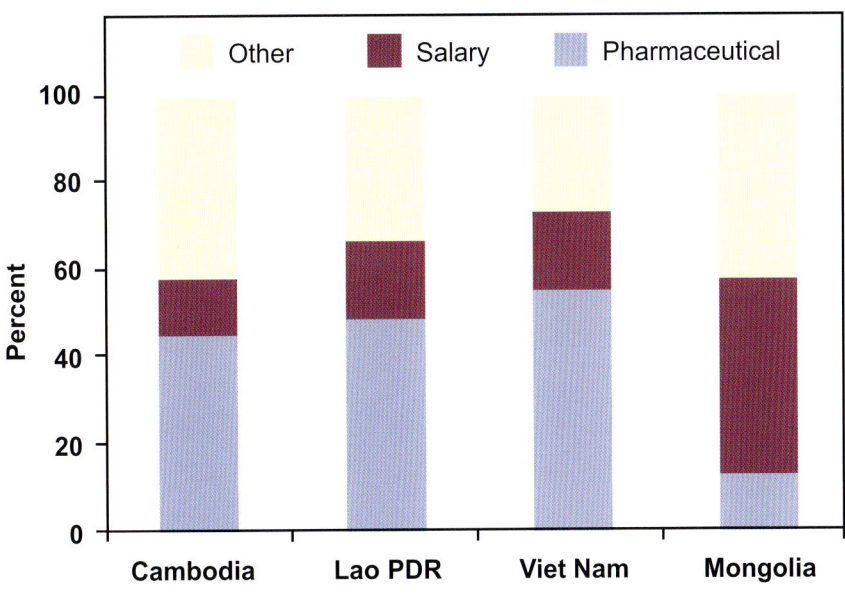

Figure 7. Components of health expenditure (2005)

Source: Midterm review of implementation: Regional Strategy on Health Care Financing in the WHO Western Pacific Region 2006-2010, P. Annear, 31 August 2008

it can comprise a large share of total health expenditures and create a major out-of-pocket burden for the sick and poor.

Pharmaceutical and diagnostic expenses account for about half of total health spending in Cambodia, China, the Lao People's Democratic Republic and Viet Nam. These countries also have high out-of-pocket payments (Figure 8), reflecting the fact that charges for pharmaceuticals and diagnostics comprise a major part of the salaries of providers. The inverse was found in Mongolia, where pharmaceuticals account for only 12% of total expenditures and out-of-pocket payments are 28%.

Many ministries of health in the Asia Pacific region have weak financial management capacities and play little role in deciding the overall budgetary allocation to the health sector. Ministries of finance, economic planning and investment dominate this process. The roles of central and local governments in health care financing have radically changed, especially where public

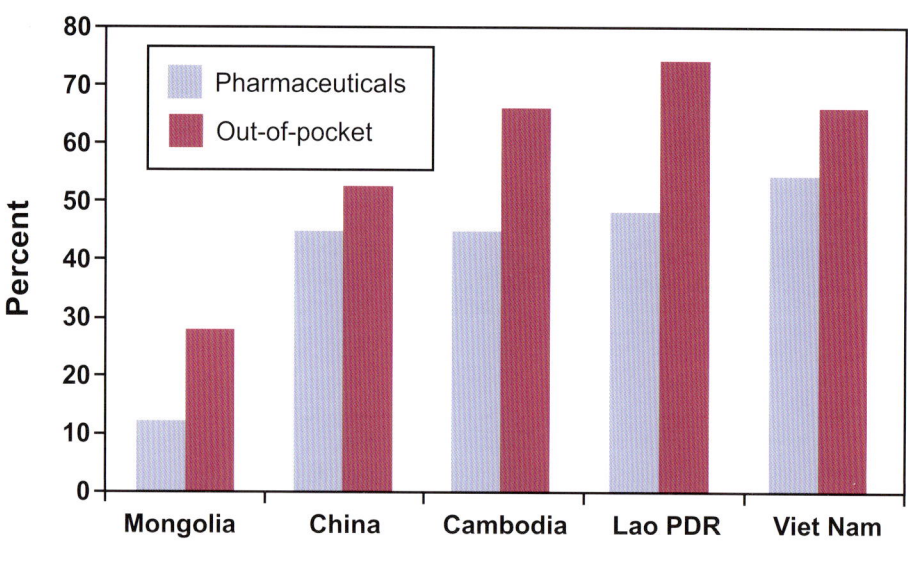

Figure 8. Components of health expenditure (2005)

Source: Midterm review of implementation: Regional Strategy on Health Care Financing in the WHO Western Pacific Region 2006-2010, P. Annear, 31 August 2008

sector reform has included decentralization. Difficulties have been created in monitoring allocation, disbursement and utilization of financial resources at different levels. Central governments bear chief responsibility for national health programmes, but often have little information on subnational health budgets.

Local governments in developing countries often have limited means of mobilizing enough financial resources for local needs. Resource-poor geographical regions face challenges in ensuring equitable distribution and use of resources, including central government subsidies. In Papua New Guinea, actual health spending deviates from initial plans due to delayed financial allocation, and slow and delayed budget disbursement is also reported. Such spending patterns affect planning and budget cycles, making it more difficult to provide quality health care and can also increase household health payments.

3. Health financing for universal coverage

Universal coverage is the most important objective in health systems financing. It is achieved when all people have access to a full range of needed personal and preventive health services of adequate quality, without excessive financial burden. In the Asia Pacific region, all governments are committed to ensuring good quality health care to their populations at affordable costs.

3.1 Universal coverage is difficult to achieve if OOP payments are greater than 30% of THE

Global experience with different systems of health financing allow comparisons of various approaches on how best to achieve universal coverage, especially for the poor and vulnerable. Evidence suggests that a strong public role in health financing, whether through payroll or general taxes, is essential for health systems to protect the poor.[15] Evidence also demonstrates that health systems with the strongest state role are likely the most equitable and achieve better aggregate health outcomes.[16,17]

Low- and middle-income countries, in which government expenditures on health are low, tend to have high shares of out-of-pocket payments, such as user fees and other direct private payments without reimbursements. It appears difficult to achieve universal coverage if out-of-pocket payments exceed 30% of total health expenditures. Out-of-pocket payments create substantial financial barriers in accessing health care, and low-income households

---

[15] Gilson L, et al. Challenging inequity through health systems. Final report. Knowledge Network on Health Systems. 2007. WHO Commission on the Social Determinants of Health.

[16] Rannan-Eliya R, Somanathan A. Equity in health and health care systems in Asia. In: The Elgar companion to health economics. Jones AM, editor. Cheltenham: Edward Elgar; 2006.

[17] Mackintosh M, Koivusalo M. Health systems and commercialisation: In search of good sense. Commercialisation of health care: Global and local dynamics and policy responses. In: Mackintosh M, Koivusalo M, . Basingstoke: Palgrave; 2005.

frequently face catastrophic health costs when out-of-pocket payments are more than 30% of total health expenditures. Global data illustrating this relationship are shown in Figure 9. A similar relationship is found for rates of household impoverishment and the share of OOP spending on health.

Most OECD countries achieved universal coverage while limiting out-of-pocket payments to 20%–30% of total health expenditures.[18] However, out-of-pocket payments cannot be an absolute health financing indicator for universal coverage. High out-of-pocket payments are found in some OECD countries such as Mexico, the Republic of Korea and Switzerland, or in developing countries such as Malaysia and Thailand, which have achieved near-universal coverage. Out-of-pocket payments in these countries are mainly contributed by co-payments under their insurance policies or by high-income groups, which can afford to use private providers.[19] Therefore, the main components and reasons for high out-of-pocket payments and their impact on coverage and access among low- income and vulnerable people must be studied when governments formulate health financing strategies to reduce out-of-pocket payments.

3.2 Universal coverage is difficult to achieve if public financing is less than 5% of GDP

Global data suggest that the levels of catastrophic and impoverishing expenditures are low when there is general government spending on health at levels of 5%–6% of GDP (Figure 10.) Higher government spending generally provides adequate public infrastructure and health service delivery at subsidized cost. Therefore, there is less need to consume health services in the private sector, where OOP payments are usually required at the point of service delivery. The opposite is true if government expenditures on health are low. Access and equity become a critical issue when out-of-pocket payments dominate.

---

[18] Elizabeth Docteur and Howard Oxley. Health-Care Systems: Lessons from the Reform Experience. OECD Working Papers, 2003.

[19] Bonu, S. I. Bhushan, and D. Peters. 2007. Incidence, Intensity, and Correlates of Catastrophic Out-of-Pocket Health Payments in India. Economics and Research Department Working Papers Series 102. ADB Manila.

Public financing, mainly through taxation or social health insurance or a combination of the two, is the dominant form of prepayment financing in countries that have achieved near universal coverage. Tax-based and social health insurance financing have comparative advantages and disadvantages, but both provide the risk pooling and cross-subsidization which are essential for universal coverage, access and financial protection.[20] Mixed health financing arrangements with some type of taxation, prepayment contributions, co-payments, user fees, targeted subsidies and other safety net components can provide good coverage and equal access. It is crucial that health financing in developing countries does not affect access and utilization of health services among the poor and vulnerable. Health financing must not expose low-income households to impoverishment. The level of public financing must be sufficient to provide at least a basic package of necessary health services and protect low-income households from catastrophic health expenditures.[21,22,23]

3.3 Fiscal space, aid effectiveness and efficiency gains

Low government health expenditures are a roadblock to universal coverage. The WHO Commission on Macroeconomics and Health estimated that the minimum expenditure for scaling up a set of essential interventions, including for the poor, was about US$ 34 per capita in 2001. However, this can be as much as US$ 100 if health system inefficiencies are taken into account.[24,25] The challenge lies in both augmenting public resources for health and using resources more efficiently.

---

[20] Technical Briefs for Policy-Makers. Achieving Universal Health Coverage: Developing Health Financing Systems.

[21] *Investing in Health WHO Commission on Macroeconomics and Health Final Report.* 2003

[22] Costing exercises for achieving the health MDGs in Cambodia, and studies in other low income countries have confirmed the validity of the $35-$100 estimates.

[23] Out-of-pocket health expenditure and debt in poor households: evidence from Cambodia. van Damme, W. Leemput, L. van, Por, I., Hardeman, W., Meessen, B. *Tropical Medicine & International Health Volume 9 Issue 2*, Pages 273 – 280 Published Online: 3 Feb 2004

[24] Investing in Health WHO Commission on Macroeconomics and Health Final Report. 2003

[25] Costing exercises for achieving the health MDGs in Cambodia, and studies in other low income countries have confirmed the validity of the $35-$100 estimates..

Figure 9. Percentage of households with catastrophic expenditures vs. share of out-of-pocket payment in total health expenditure

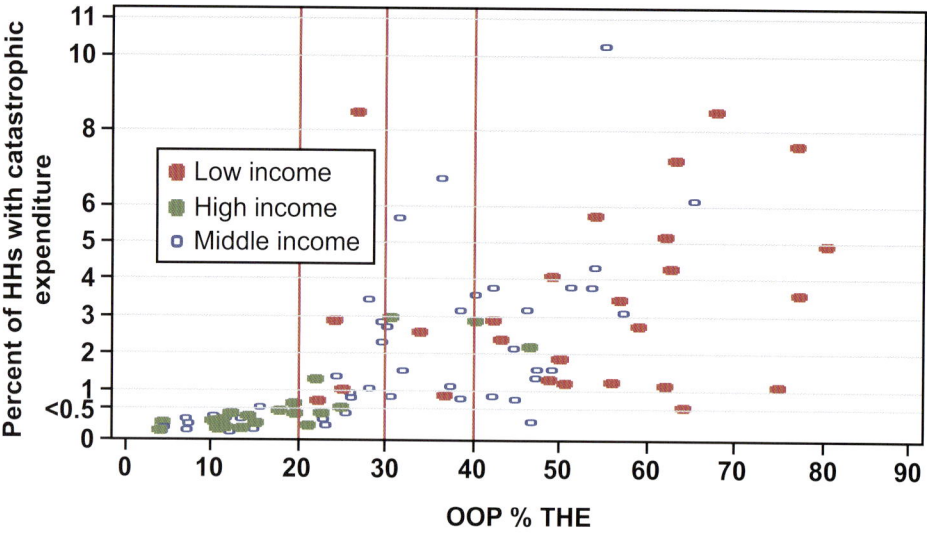

Source: K Xu, et. al. Protecting households from catastrophic health spending. Health Affairs, 26. No. 4 (2007): 972-983

Figure 10. Percentage of households with catastrophic expenditures vs. government health expenditures as a share of GDP

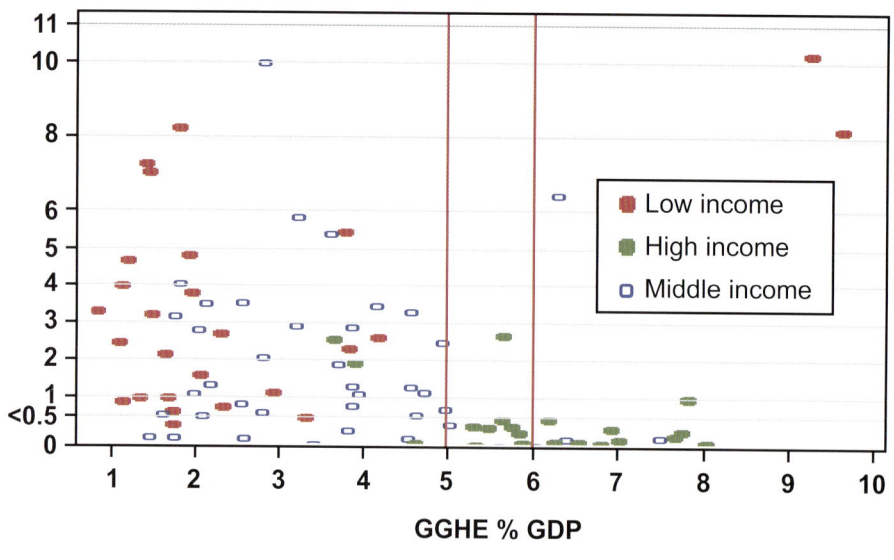

GDPSource: KXu, DB Evans, K Kawabata, et al. (2003): Household catastrophic health expenditure: a multi-country analysis. The Lancet. Vol(362):111-117

Regional data suggest that with the exception of some Pacific island countries, tax revenues in the Asia Pacific region—13.2% of GDP, with total government revenues at 16.6 % of GDP[26]—are the lowest of any region in the world. This suggests that there is room to raise revenues to finance a higher level of spending as a percentage of GDP, especially in countries experiencing economic growth.

Increasing budgetary room for health without compromising a government's financial position is at the core of health financing efforts. Broad fiscal approaches to increase health spending in this region might include increasing domestic tax revenues, expanding the tax base, developing social health insurance, borrowing externally or seeking debt repayment relief.

Aid effectiveness, including alignment and harmonization of overseas development assistance (ODA) with national priorities, is an important issue in the region. The mean level of ODA in the region is only about 11% of health expenditures, but it is much higher in some low-income countries.

Therefore, countries should exert efforts to increase ODA for the health sector and at the same time to improve the effectiveness of aid.[27]

Improving the efficient use of all resources available to governments is feasible. Public expenditure primarily needs a focus on national health goals, particularly the needs of the poor as well as improvements in public sector performance at all levels. Better allocative, technical and distributional use of resources, as well as results-based management, can improve efficiency.

Separation of government financing and provision of health services through engagement of the private sector might be an option in countries where the private sector plays an important role in service provision. National health efforts could also include the non-state private sector as a useful resource for health if regulatory and quality standards can be met.

---

[26] Global Health Disparities: the role of health financing, donor assistance, and human resources. CGFNS Symposium Philadelphia, December 2007 Marko Vujicic The World Bank

[27] Fiscal Space for Health: Use of Donor Assistance. Dr. P Gottret, South Asia Region The World Bank, Colombo, March 18, 2009

3.4 Health systems strengthening and health financing

Health financing must be placed in the context of an overall health systems apporach that leads to universal coverage. The WHO framework for action for strengthening health systems to improve health outcomes identified six health system building blocks, one of which is health financing as shown in Figure 11.

Health financing plays a central role in the process of achieving overall health systems goals to improve equity, risk protection and efficiency. There are key links and dynamic interactions between health financing and the other system building blocks. These include:

3.4.1 Service delivery

Health financing policies need to secure an agreed benefit package to address national health needs, especially those of the poor and including all types of care: preventive, promotive, curative and rehabilitative. Allocative, technical

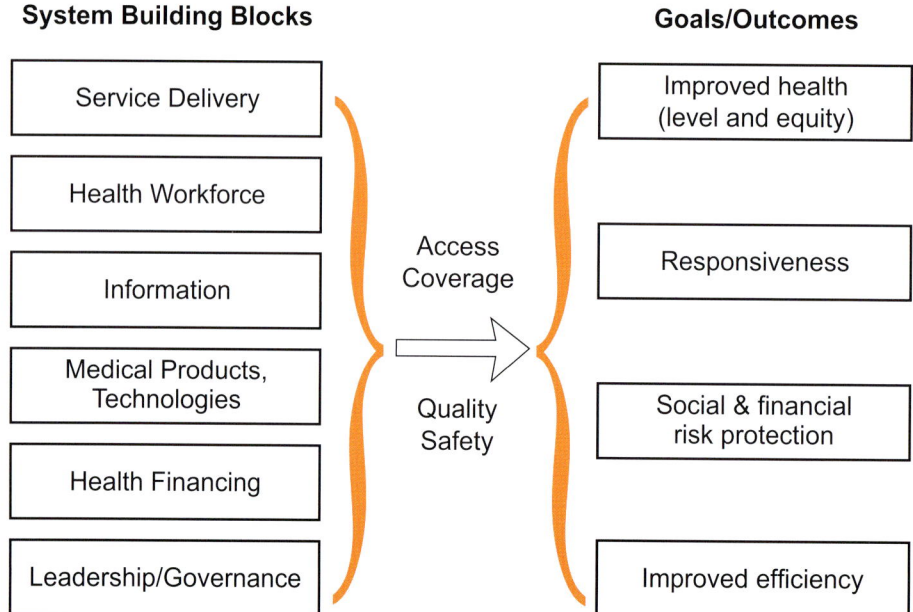

Figure 11. Health Systems framework with six building blocks

and distributional efficiencies in health financing could contribute significantly to systems gains from better structure, organization and management, as well as cost-effectiveness of service delivery. Health financing must provide incentives that encourage quality of services.

3.4.2 Health workforce

Health systems are highly labour intensive, and compensation of health workers comprises a large part of health expenditures in most countries. Various provider payment methods incorporated in financing mechanisms need to be effectively used to increase health workforce motivation. These could influence the health workforce skill mix to deliver priority health services, deployment, retention and performance in underserved areas. They could also be used to effectively engage the private sector in the national health agenda.

3.4.3 Health information

Health financing and expenditure information that is reliably disaggregated, in conjunction with epidemiological and health outcomes data, is necessary to support policies and technical reviews. Data needs include sources of funds, use of health service providers by beneficiaries among different population groups, and the extent of financial health protection in terms of population health coverage, catastrophic payment incidence and poverty impacts.

3.4.4 Medical products and technologies

Expenditure on medicines and medical products constitutes the largest share of out-of-pocket payments in the Asia Pacific region. Evidence suggests that more than half of medical product use is irrational use. Health financing policy, together with medicines policies, could reduce this significantly.

3.4.5 Leadership and governance

Good governance and leadership are needed to increase public spending on health and to maintain the focus on the attainment of universal coverage.

The leadership and governance functions need legislative and regulatory frameworks that support prepayment and risk pooling arrangements, and rationalize health spending both in the public and private sectors. Leadership is needed to make health care financing more accountable to the public, particularly in regards to illicit payments.

4. Health Financing Strategy for the Asia Pacific Region (2010–2015)

4.1 Advancing towards universal coverage

This Strategy is meant to assist Member States achieve universal coverage through effective health financing. The diagram below is a schematic presentation of the Strategy.

An increase in financial resources to health and greater efficiency in use of resources will allow expansion of services, especially for primary health care. More prepayment, risk-pooling and effective social protection will allow extension of services, especially the poor and other vulnerable populations, as well as reduce out-of-pocket payments. These dimensions call for targeted interventions suited to each country in the following eight strategic areas:

(1) increasing investment and public spending on health
(2) improving aid effectiveness for health
(3) improving efficiency by rationalizing health expenditures
(4) increasing the use of prepayment and risk-pooling

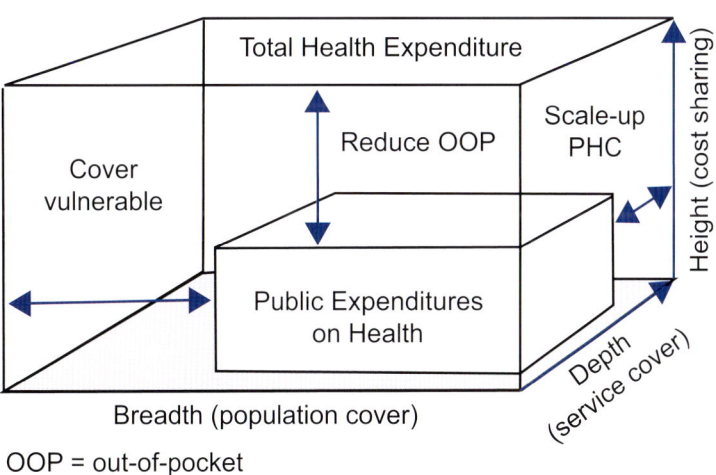

Figure 12. Attainment of universal coverage

OOP = out-of-pocket
PHC = primary health care

(5) improving provider payment methods
(6) strengthening safety-net mechanisms for the poor and vulnerable
(7) improving evidence and information for policymaking
(8) improving monitoring and evaluation of policy changes.

The draft Strategy adds three areas of emphasis that are not in the existing Strategy on Health Care Financing for Countries of the Western Pacific and South-East Asia Regions (2006–2010). They are: (1) improving aid effectiveness; (2) improving efficiency by rationalizing health expenditures; and (3) improving provider payment methods.

The following diagram shows how full implementation will be progressively and incrementally achieved. Financing progresses from private, out-of-pocket payments to prepaid and risk-pooled schemes. Eventually, the pooled funding is sufficient to finance universal coverage.

4.2   Goals and targets

The goal of this Strategy is to help countries attain universal coverage that ensures access to quality health services for better health outcomes. Evidence

Figure 13. Steps towards universal coverage

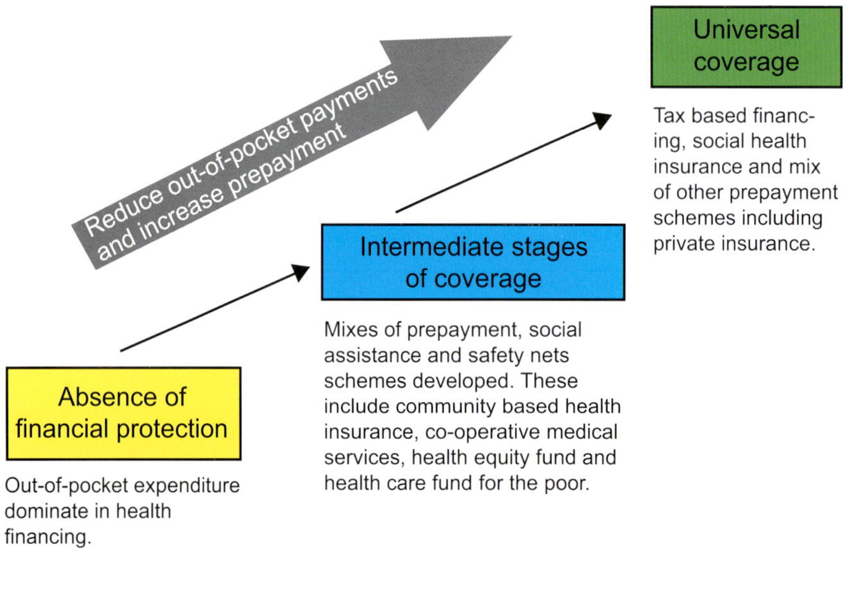

Figure 14. Links between health financing strategy and health outcomes

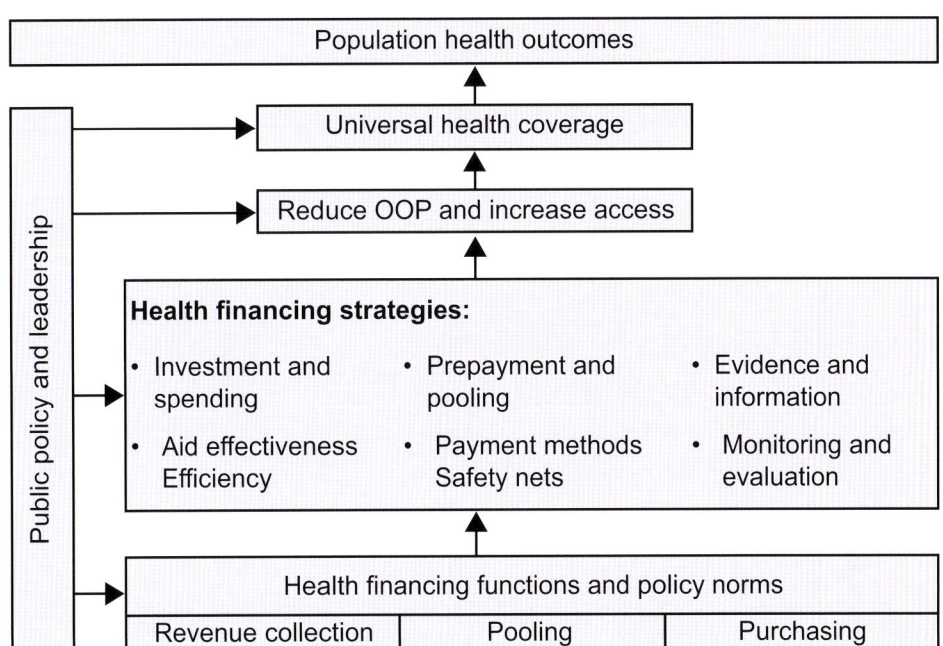

suggests that universal coverage is more likely in countries where public financing of health, including tax financing and social health insurance, is around 5% of GDP. This is an important goal for all countries in the Asia Pacific region, which aim to attain universal coverage. There are exceptions, with some countries attaining near universal coverage at lower levels of public spending on health. Other countries are still in the early stages of universal coverage, although their level of health spending is relatively high. Therefore, the Strategy encourages countries to set their own realistic targets with a clear strategic course of action to increase public spending and its share in total health expenditures.

The following targets are proposed to monitor and evaluate progress:
- out-of-pocket (OOP) spending should not exceed 30%–40% of total health expenditure;
- total health expenditure should be at least 4%–5% of GDP;
- over 90% population is covered by prepayment and risk-pooling schemes; and

- close to 100% coverage of vulnerable populations with social assistance and safety-net programmes.

4.3 Supportive environment for health financing reforms

Implementation of the Strategy will need strong commitment and active engagement from all stakeholders, both within and outside the health sector. A supportive and enabling environment would need to include:

(1) Consensus on and commitment to universal coverage, including:
   (a) multisectoral and multi-stakeholder consensus on the goals;
   (b) commitment to roles and responsibilities in achieving universal coverage for all;
   (c) availability of evidence on the impact of public investments in health;
   (d) forums for disseminating policy analyses for high-level advocacy, particularly with ministries of health and financing; and
   (e) plans to address the concerns of stakeholders who may be opposed.

(2) Development and implementation of policy, including:
   (a) technical capacity to generate information and formulate policy;
   (b) capacity to review and enforce legislation and regulation; and
   (c) administrative and management capacity at national and subnational levels.

(3) Transparency and accountability in all processes, including
   (a) resource management;
   (b) monitoring and evaluation of policy; and
   (c) carrying out designated roles and responsibilities.

Actions within the Strategy should be guided by health financing policy norms relative to the three main health financing functions of revenue collection, revenue pooling and purchasing of services.

4.4 Strategic areas for action in health financing for universal coverage

4.4.1 Strategic Area 1: Increasing investment and public spending on health.

Area 1 addresses the importance of appropriate levels of health spending, particularly in times of economic and financial crises. Adequate public financing is promoted as the most effective health financing mechanism to promote equity. The strategic actions include:

(1) Increase government commitment evidenced by appropriate policy development, targets, and medium- and long-term action plans.

(2) Analyse, cost and plan the investment needs of the health system for achieving universal coverage.

(3) Achieve multisectoral synergy through integrated planning with health-related sectors, the non-state sector and global programmes.

(4) Strengthen national and subnational capacities for resource mobilization, including both domestic and international options.

(5) Build and disseminate evidence on the impact of public investment in health on health outcomes, social and overall development, particularly between ministries of health and finance and planning.

4.4.2 Strategic Area 2: Improving aid effectiveness for health.

Domestic financing of health systems based on pooling and high public contributions is the best financing choice However, external aid will continue to play an important complementary role, especially in low-income countries. Area 2 promotes the efficient and effective use of aid in ways that contribute to sustainable universal coverage. This is consistent with the five pillars of the Paris Aid Declaration. The strategic actions include:

(1) Request overseas development assistance (ODA) based on a results-oriented strategic resource plan, emphasizing efforts to increase domestic financing, especially the government health budget.

(2) Use national plans to reduce fragmentation and better align ODA with the national health agenda and national coordination processes.

(3) Increase effectiveness of ODA by minimizing transaction costs and increasing the proportion that supports health in line with the general government budget.

(4) Work with all partners to increase aid predictability and reduce aid volatility.

(5) Implement simple and shared monitoring mechanisms that increase transparency and timeliness of information.

4.4.3 Strategic Area 3: Improving efficiency by rationalizing health expenditures.

Area 3 encourages achieving better value for money by rationalizing health expenditures. Both domestic and external resources should be focused on health outcomes while addressing inequity, inefficiency and low quality. The core strategic actions include:

(1) National and subnational planning processes are guided by the priorities of improving health outcomes and achieving universal coverage through appropriate balanced allocations between primary, secondary and tertiary care.

(2) Costing and cost-effectiveness analysis, medium-term expenditure frameworks (MTEF), public health expenditure reviews (PER), results-based financing (RBF), and other appropriate tools will be used to increase the efficiency of public spending.

(3) Upgrade skills critical to achieving effective use of resources, including management of health workers and service delivery, financing and regulation of the health sector. Unofficial fees and other leakages will be discouraged. Cost-effective initiatives, such as home-based care, will be promoted.

(4) Ensure timely, efficient and equitable allocation of resources to primary health care and other essential services, ensuring coverage of the poor and vulnerable and remote and underserved areas.

(5) Reduce costs of pharmaceutical supply and distribution, especially in the private sector, by implementing policies on the rational use of essential drugs, creating incentives for good prescription practices, weakening monopolies where they raise costs, and improving social marketing to reduce irrational demand for drugs and diagnostics.

(6) Engage the non-state sector in rationalizing health expenditures to attain universal coverage and strengthen primary health care.

4.4.4 Strategic Area 4: Increasing the use of prepayment and risk-pooling

Area 4 aims to increase prepayment and risk-pooling arrangements to improve equity, access and protection against the financial risks of ill-health. Strategic actions to increase population coverage by risk-pooling prepayment arrangements include:

(1) Define appropriate prepayment options, including social health insurance, with equitable contributions and benefits and develop feasible policy, targets and action plans.

(2) Advocate, raise awareness and build consensus for universal access through a mixed system of financing among all stakeholders, policy- and decision-makers, service providers and the health workforce, and consumers.

(3) Increase government commitment to effective prepayment and pooling.

(4) Implement action plans to increase population coverage and access through a combination of taxation, social health insurance and other prepayment mechanisms.

(5) Implement measures to improve efficiency and performance supported by standards and norms, legislative and accreditation instruments in both the public and private sector.

4.4.5 Strategic Area 5: Improving provider payment methods.

Area 5 focuses on provider payments as a key purchasing mechanism to influence provider and consumer behaviour and improve health systems performance. Provider payments can be used to direct the mix of the delivery of services, contain costs on the supply side and modify consumer demand. This can contribute to efficiency and improve the focus on the desired level and type of care in line with a primary health care approach. Provider payments may provide incentive options for effective engagement of the private sector. Combined with appropriate contracting, provider payments may be used to improve performance in both the public and private sectors. The strategic actions include:

(1) Evaluate current provider payment methods and their impact on health systems and financing.

(2) Examine the evidence on each payment option with respect to its potential to better match service delivery with policy goals, contain costs, decrease catastrophic spending and decrease perverse provider incentives.

(3) Review the incentives under provider payment with respect to effectively engaging the private sector.

(4) Support policy implementation with necessary legislative and regulation authority, including safeguarding the interests of the poor.

(5) Include provider payment methods in gathering, monitoring and evaluating services.

4.4.6 Strategic Area 6: Strengthening safety-net mechanisms for the poor and vulnerable

Social safety-net mechanisms aim to increase social protection by reducing barriers that exclude the poor and vulnerable from accessing health services. The barriers may be economic, political, social and cultural, or a complex interaction of all these factors. Health financing oriented towards the poor aims to eliminate financial barriers to care by reducing out-of-pocket payments and promoting pooling that provides subsidized access for the poor. Actions to advance social protection and safety-net mechanisms include:

(1) Generate and analyse evidence on the financial and social determinants of health.

(2) Ensure that planned safety-net mechanisms such as fee exemptions and premium subsidies are fully funded. Funding channels may include general taxation, earmarked taxes, cross-subsidized SHI, ODA, and voluntary contributions from the private sector, e.g. corporate social responsibility.

(3) Target subsidies to address the needs of specific vulnerable groups or particular social goals, such as maternal health care for neglected minorities or female empowerment.

(4) Strengthen the legal and regulatory framework to safeguard the needs of the poor in established financing mechanisms.

(5) Regularly monitor and evaluate the financial and social protection status of the poor and vulnerable.

4.4.7 Strategic Area 7: Improving evidence and information for policy-making

Area 7 recognizes evidence and information as the cornerstones of decision-making and policy. Appropriate quality data needs to be incorporated into routine health information systems. Actions needed to strengthen evidence-based policy include:

(1) Take stock of available evidence and identifying data and quality gaps.

(2) Develop research capacity to provide on-going evidence and information needs.

(3) Establish centres of international quality that could anchor the generation, analysis and dissemination of policy-related evidence.

(4) Strengthen capacity to use tools and techniques for policy analyses, including impact assessments using cost data, economic evaluations at the macro level, and appropriate use of epidemiological information.

(5) Strengthen capacity to improve financial management for policy through budgeting and resource tracking tools such as national health accounts and medium-term expenditure frameworks.

4.4.8 Strategic Area 8: Improving monitoring and evaluation of policy changes

The draft Health Financing Strategy for the Asia Pacific Region (2010–2015) is intended to guide future health financing work and health systems strengthening in the Asia Pacific region. Policies, interventions and strategic actions will need to be specific and relevant to each country. Area 8 calls for monitoring and evaluating progress in implementation at the regional and national levels. Monitoring indicators should be politically relevant, technically useful and kept to an essential minimum number. There are advantages to the adoption of a uniform set of indicators so progress can be compared across the region. Needed actions include:

(1) Identify information requirements, gaps in managerial and analytical skills, and sources of funding for monitoring and evaluation of policy.

(2) Undertake capacity-building in the areas of economic principles for health policy monitoring and evaluation.

(3) Integrate health financing indicators into an overall health monitoring and evaluation framework. The focus is on equity, efficiency, coverage, access and a reduction in out-of-pocket payments.

(4) Encourage participatory monitoring and evaluation, including as many stakeholders as possible.

(5) Link monitoring and evaluation to policy review by providing timely reports to health planners.

5. Conclusions

The draft Health Financing Strategy for the Asia Pacific Region (2010–2015) supports universal coverage and access to quality health services for improved health outcomes in the Asia Pacific region. It is driven by country-level initiatives, actions and findings from regional health financing assessments, a changing global environment, an increasing body of evidence and emphasis on a primary health care approach in health systems strengthening to achieve universal coverage.

Universal coverage aims to improve the health status of the poor and vulnerable, especially women and children. Attaining universal coverage requires urgent government attention and action. For the most part, those countries that have been most successful in protecting the poor and vulnerable and in achieving the greatest health gains for the resources available are those that have had long-term commitments to primary health care, universal coverage and social health protection.

The draft Health Financing Strategy for the Asia Pacific Region (2010–2015) can be used as a guide by WHO and Member States to accelerate progress towards universal coverage. It advocates substantial reductions in out-of-pocket payments, which remain both the single main cause of household impoverishment and a financial barrier in accessing health services. The Strategy calls on governments to increase public spending on health and strengthen safety-net mechanisms to ensure greater coverage and access to subsidized care, especially for the poor. The Strategy also underlines inefficiencies in resource use and provides guidance on strategies to increase both the efficiency and effectiveness of health services.

Universal coverage is an ambitious goal. But progress towards universal coverage has been demonstrated to be feasible in both the short and long term. The Strategy encourages each country to examine its own health financing situation and take actions leading to a higher level of health by improving coverage, financial protection, and health systems. The Strategy will guide countries in these efforts to provide comprehensive and quality health services for all, including those presently underserved. Such efforts will improve the quality of life throughout the Asia Pacific region.

Health Financing Strategy Glossary

Access	Ability to utilize available health services without any significant barriers or obstacles
Aid effectiveness	The effectiveness of development aid in achieving economic or human development (or development targets).
Allocative efficiency	Resources are distributed among multiple activities within a sector or programme in a way that maximizes a specified outcome.
Capitation payment	A fixed amount of money per patient per unit of time is paid in advance to a provider for the delivery of health care services. The amount is determined mainly by the range of services provided. Controls use of health care resources by putting the provider at financial risk for services provided.
Catastrophic health expenditure	Cumulative expenses on health care that exceed 40% of non-food household expenditures.
Community-based health insurance (CBHI)	Small-scale voluntary social insurance. Typically a local health centre contracts with CBHI scheme to provide services. Seen as a step towards wider SHI coverage.
Co-payment	A proportion of total billed costs of services paid at the time of service by insured patients, mainly used as a cost-control measure.
Coverage	Coverage of a population for health services often represented in three dimensions: breadth, or the extent of the covered population; depth, or the types of services covered; and height, or the level of cost sharing.
Diagnostic-related groups	Form of payment per one classified group of similar medical interventions expected to have similar hospital resource use.
Effectiveness	The degree to which objectives are achieved and the extent to which targeted problems are resolved. In contrast to efficiency, effectiveness is determined without reference to costs.
Evidence	Scientifically valid and unbiased information that can be used for making policies.

Excess or deductible amount	The portion of a claim that is not covered by the insurance provider. It is the amount of expenses that must be paid out of pocket before the benefits of the policy can apply.
Fee for service	Payment to a provider for the cost of services provided, usually at the time of service.
Financial burden	The amount a household pays for health care relative to its income or relative to its capacity to pay.
Financial protection	Ultimate effect of health financing schemes that eliminate or greatly reduce the amounts patients must pay out of pocket.
Fiscal space	Room in government budget that allows it to provide resources for a desired purpose without jeopardizing the sustainability of its financial position or the stability of the economy.
Gross Domestic Product	Gross Domestic Product, the total value of goods and services produced in a country, usually within a year.
Global budget	Form of payment to finance health services by a lump-sum allocation, leaving decisions about how it is used to decentralized management.
Global economic crisis or recession	An economic downturn that is felt in many countries at the same time, with job losses in producer countries due to decreased lending and purchasing power in developed countries.
Government health expenditures	Defined as governmental inputs to health financing from all levels. It may also include social health insurance and external aid, in which case "public financing" is a better term.
Health equity	Defined alternatively as equal health status for different income groups, equal access to care, equal payment for health care, equal uptake of public subsidy, etc.
Health equity funds	A targeted subsidy used for paying part of hospital and other healthcare costs for the poor.
Health outcomes	Population health status that includes infant and child mortality rates, life expectancy at birth, maternal mortality rates

Insurance benefits	The package of health services that members of the insurance scheme are entitled to.
Medium-term expenditure framework	A mode of budget planning referring to the expenditures for the present financial year and the two following years, that encourages cooperation across ministries and planning over a longer horizon than usual.
Millennium Development Goals	Eight goals range from halving extreme poverty to halting the spread of HIV/AIDS and providing universal primary education, all by the target date of 2015. Three of them are related directly to health outcomes. They form a blueprint agreed to by all countries and the world's leading development institutions.
National health accounts (NHA)	A data base system that provides information on financial resources used for health, their sources, and the way they are used. It allows monitoring trends in health spending for public and private sectors, different health care activities, providers, diseases, population groups and regions.
NCMS	New Cooperative Medical Scheme, a voluntary health insurance system covering nearly all rural residents in China with government subsidy.
ODA	Overseas Development Assistance represents foreign aid and assistance coming from donor to recipient countries.
Out-of-pocket expenditure	Costs for health care that are paid by individuals at the time of treatment through user fees, co-payments and direct payments for example for medicine.
Paris Aid Declaration	International agreement endorsed in 2005 in which over 100 ministers, heads of aid agencies, and other senior officials committed their countries and organizations to increase efforts in harmonization, alignment and managing aid for results with a set of monitorable actions and indicators.
Pay-for-performance (P4P)	Transfer of money or material goods conditional on taking a measurable action or achieving a predetermined performance target. Some times it refers to result-based financing.

People-centered health systems	It refers where health system support people's right and duty to participate in making decisions about their health care, not only in issues of treatment, but for broader issues of health care planning and implementation
Poverty level	A level of income defined in terms of the costs of basic nutritional food. The current international poverty level is US$ 1.25 per day.
Prioritization	Operating within a limited budget for health, governments indicate their priorities by increasing spending on the health services they value the most.
Provider payments	The way that health care providers are paid for delivering health services. Fee-for-service, capitation, salary, and global budget are common provider payment methods.
Public expenditure reviews	Public expenditure reviews analyse the allocation and management of public expenditure. They can be used to inform strategic planning and budget preparation and to identify ways in which to improve efficiency and effectiveness.
Public health expenditures	Includes government health budget disbursements and other "public" sources such as social health insurance and external donor aid.
Purchasing of services	One of the functions of health financing and health governance bodies. Two alternatives are directly owning health facilities and employing health staff, or paying an independent entity to provide a package of services to a given population.
Results-based budgeting	Budget process in which programme formulation revolves around a set of predefined objectives and expected results; and expected results justify the resource requirements which are derived from outputs to achieve the results.
Results-based financing	Results-Based Financing (RBF) can help governments achieve national health goals by organising their health systems differently. The emphasis is shifted from distributing and using resources to achieving results.
Retrospective reimbursement	Reimbursement paid after a period of time to a patient for a payment made for health services.

Risk-pooling	Pooling health risks among young, healthy people, and older and more illness-prone people in an insurance scheme in order to lower the average financial risk to the insurer.
Social health insurance	Insurance scheme providing a defined package of health benefits, usually compulsory for all workers, with premiums based only based on wages.
Social marketing	Planning and implementation of programs designed to bring about social change using concepts from commercial marketing.
Social safety net mechanisms	Services provided by the state, such as welfare, unemployment benefit, universal healthcare and other subsidies, which prevent individuals from falling into poverty beyond a certain level.
Technical efficiency	A fixed level of resources is used in ways for a single activity that maximizes a specified output; similar to productivity.
Total health expenditures	The sum of private spending on health, government health budgets, and other sources of financing such as social health insurance. This will then include personal health care, collective health services and the operation of health systems, plus capital investment.
Universal coverage	Nearly all people have access to good quality needed services without facing catastrophic financial expenses.